HOW TO REDUCE BREASTS NATURALLY WITHOUT SURGERY.

TIFFANY HILLS.

TABLE OF CONTENTS

INTRODUCTION

Breasts are of different shapes and sizes, too big, big, too small and weird. Studies have shown that good looking boobs attracts opposite sex even same sex as well. The social pressure of having a perfect body and good boobs can weigh heavy on ladies. That is why most female celebrities try to maintain perfect size, natural and gorgeous boobs as role models. According to a popular celebrity "sex is not enough, I have learnt one major beauty lessons that good boobs and curves can make men go haywire". There are no right or wrong. No doubt, people are more concern about breasts enlargement or how to have firmer breasts

without surgery and less concern on maintaining an average size in order to reduce breast cancer risk and other illness.

Reasons why a person may want to reduce breast size are:-

(a). for cosmetic or psychological reasons.

(b). Age.

(c). Hormonal changes due to medications, pregnancy or thyroid issues can also have an impact.

The pains and costs of going through surgery can be discouraging hence there are natural ways to reduce breast size without surgery.

Reports have shown that women with bigger boobs are bullied and body shamed daily, some easily sick of neck, shoulder and back pains due to heaviness of the breast. This book is written to show you how to reduce your breasts without surgery, simple self-help procedures.

Breasts contain mostly fats, so a strategy that reduces overall body fats may work well.

The right method for reducing breast size depends on a person's overall health. Breast development occurs throughout a woman's life. Some women may consider large breasts to be a cosmetic advantage. However, large breasts can also associated with many ailments, including shoulder, back and neck pains.

The breast is composed of adipose tissue and glandular tissue bound to hormone receptors. Adipose tissue is the fatty tissue that fills the breast, while glandular tissue, or mammary tissue, is responsible for milk production. Hormonal changes in the body over time can cause this tissue to expand, resulting in larger breasts.

HOW TO REDUCE BREASTS SIZE NATURALLY.

1. EXERCISES.

Exercise can help you lose body fat, which also helps to reduce breast size over time.

Targeted exercise can burn fats, push-ups and other chest exercises will support the arm and chest muscles directly to remove fats from the breasts themselves.

Cardiovascular exercises that increase a person's heart rate are highly effective at burning fats throughout the body. How to reduce your breast size with exercise depends on how you engage on the health and fitness factors known to

be the best breast reduction
exercises.

Best Exercises to Lose Breasts are:-

1. Jogging

All types of aerobic exercise help reduce body fat, including chest fat. So walk, jog, run, or ride a bike to make your breasts smaller.

Duration

20 to 40 minutes

2. Push-ups

Push-ups help tone, reduce size, and improve the appearance of your chest and pectoral muscles (pectoralis major).

5 to 10 minutes

3. Swimming

The actions you perform while swimming strengthen your chest and shoulder muscles, tone your pectoral muscles, and help improve the appearance of your chest.

Duration

10 to 20 minutes

4. Yoga

Practicing yoga poses such as Prayer Pose, Crescent Pose and Frog Pose can reduce breast size and give firmness.

Duration

Yoga pose for 10-20 seconds.

Yoga Poses for Natural Breast Reduction

Back pain and discomfort are common when breast enlargement occurs. You can follow the breast reduction treatments outlined in this article, but yoga can help speed up the process. Certain yoga poses can help firm your breasts, improve firmness and reduces size.

These regular exercises can help reduce breast size easily:-

1. Strength training combined with a higher level of daily activity with quantified nutrition will help burn excess fat. Burning all the fat in the body will gradually help reduce acne breakouts. When people think of

losing weight, the first thing that comes to mind is cardio or strength training. In recent times, exercises have been identified as one of the secret of how to lose breast fat quickly. Try the pull-up exercise with weights, as this is the best exercise for beauties with heavy breasts. Ideally, if the goal is to lose fat, a person should burn calories and maintain muscle mass, which can be achieved by incorporating both types of exercise into their training routine, along with a healthy and low calorie diet.

2. Cardio Cardiovascular exercise burns calories and improves heart health. Strength training helps burn calories, maintain/build muscle and

keep our metabolism high. Therefore, to improve body composition and stay in shape, cardiovascular and resistance training should be incorporated into one's workout regimen while following a healthy diet. Cardiovascular exercises that help reduce chest weight includes:- jogging, shoulder pushups, side dumbbells, chest presses and wall pushups.

3. Stretching Women with heavy breasts should include stretching and range of motion exercises in their regular exercise routine to strengthen the shoulder and back muscles. It will also help eliminate

back pain and prevent the risk of muscle injury during exercise.

4. Train your deltoids. Exercising and strengthening your upper back and posterior deltoids is essential to maintaining good posture. Some good exercises to do are dumbbells or barbell exercises for the upper back and face pulls for the deltoids. Show love to your body with these exercises to reduce your bust size. So you can enjoy simple things like getting off and running without rocking the city.

Research has proven that it is possible to reduce your breast with exercise that is why most female athletes that engage in exercises regularly do not grow bigger breasts.

2. DIET.

Diet is one of the natural remedies that help to reduce breast size quickly. The breasts are mostly made up of fats or adipose tissues. Losing body fat reduces breast sizes.

People can lose body fats by losing more calories than what they eat, by eating healthy diet. A low-calorie, highly nutritious diet helps to shrink breast tissues.

Focus on eating nutrient dense foods that are low in calories. These have been proven to be one of the natural methods of reducing breast size without surgery. Vegetables, fruits, fatty fish example salmon, lean meats and grilled chicken, can help you feel good, have firmer breast while still supporting healthy weight loss.

People who are breastfeeding or pregnant should consult their doctors or midwife before trying to lose weight.

3. CHANGE BRA.

Bra cannot permanently change breast size, but bras like fruit of the loom women's front closure cotton bra or breast reduction bra can create the illusion of smaller breast. The Playtex women's18-hour ultimate lift wireless full- coverage bra can give breast good shape and make the breasts looks good, flatter and smaller on the chest.

Also bras like breast support band, posture corrector bra offers more supportive straps, which reduces neck and back pains.

Wearing a supportive, well-fitting bra can significantly improve a breast shape and comfort levels. Many online stores offer free bra-fitting services. Simply changing bras can reduce pains associated with large breasts.

4. REDUCES ESTROGEN LEVEL.

Flaxseed reduces estrogen levels. Estrogen plays vital role in the development of breast tissues. It has been proven that excess estrogen reduces breast size, most especially in people with hormonal imbalances.

Hormonal contraceptives contain progesterone and estrogen can make breasts grow bigger. The effect usually goes away once the person stops taking the medication.

According to research, estrogen levels can be reduce in the body through dietary changes.

For instance, animal studies suggest that flaxseed supplements helps to regulate estrogen levels by reducing estrogen expression in the ovaries. Flaxseeds also protect the heart, prevent inflammations and reduce the risk of having cancer.

However, there is evidence about natural remedies to reduce estrogen in the body. You can talk to your doctor about estrogen lowering medication.

5. BINDING.

Binding is the process of wrapping material tightly around the breasts to flatten them. Example post surgery breast implant stabilizer and compression band, breast augmentation reduction strap and medical breast implant stabilizer band. It does not prevent the breasts from growing or shrink breasts tissues, but it helps the breasts look smaller and may help you feel more comfortable at home, while driving or at workplace. Consult your doctor about the safest way to use a binder.

You can find binders in online stores like Amazon.com.

HOW TO REDUCE BREASTS SIZE IN 7 DAYS AT HOME.

 The best and easy exercises to reduce breast size at home:

1. Wall Press:

Wall Pressing is one of the easiest exercises you can do anywhere. All you need to get started is a wall. The process is similar to regular push-ups, except here you do it while standing. This exercise strengthens your chest muscles and burns fat in your chest and underarms. If you continue daily, you will see improvement within a week.

Steps to perform:

• **Stand facing the wall, slightly more than arm's length away from the wall.**

• **Take a comfortable position, perhaps a few inches away from a wall.**

• **Place your palms flat on the wall at shoulder height, about shoulder width apart.**

• **Stand to your feet on the ground. Do not lift or move your legs during the exercise.**

• **Next, bend your elbows and lower your upper body toward the wall.**

• **Lower yourself and count five times.**

• Breathe in and lower yourself down.

• Lower your hips gently, keep your back and hips straight.

READ: Exercises to remove underarm bra bulges

2. Push-ups:

Push-ups strengthen the chest muscles and can reduce breast size. It also tightens the area to prevent sagging. However, you cannot do miracles with push-ups alone. It must be combined with other forms of cardio and strength training to reduce body fat and produce a visible change in breast size.

Steps to perform:

• Lie flat on a rubber mat with your hands next to your shoulders. You can also do this on the floor.

• Now try pressing your body onto your knees. Then pull your stomach in. Try to keep your body in a straight line at all times.

Remain in the position for a few seconds, then press down. This push-up exercise is a great exercise to do at home to reduce breast size.

How to reduce breast size while sleeping is, lie flat and face the floor during sleep.

• In general, this is the best breast reduction with exercise.

3. Bent Knee Push-Up:

This is a modified push-up. Do the exercise with your knees bent rather than lying down. Just like a traditional push-up, bending your knees pushes you up, then strengthens and tones your pectoral muscles. This is a demanding exercise that forces you to cut your calories significantly.

How to perform:

• Lie on your stomach and place your hands under your shoulders.

• Bend your legs behind you and keep your ankles crossed.

• **Extend your arms to push your body up and slowly bend your arms and lower body toward the floor.**

4. Aerobic Exercise:

Aerobic exercise such as walking, jogging, swimming and aerobics can help you lose all body fat. You'll see a noticeable difference as it boosts your metabolism and burns calories faster. When done along with push-ups and strength training, it can change the size of your breasts and make them appear smaller but firmer.

5. Leg Raise:

The leg raise exercise is not just for reducing breast size. You can strengthen your abs and control the sagging of your chest. With this easy breast reduction exercise you can get great results without going to the gym. To learn how, follow these steps:

How to Perform:

• Lie flat on the floor with your arms at your sides.

• Squeeze your abs toward your spine.

. Straighten your knees, breathe-in and lift your legs from the floor.

• Hold your breath for a few seconds while keeping your hips on the floor. Then, exhale as you lower your feet to the floor.

• Then repeats this exercise 5-10 times. This is a great breast reduction exercise and if you do this work out regularly, your breasts will be in perfect shape.

Read: Armpit Fat Reduction Exercises

6. Shrugs:

Shrugs are arguably one of the most effective exercises for reducing cup size. Push your muscles inwards and strengthen them. Exercising regularly can make your chest look good and firmer. For shrugging, using dumbbells or using a bottle of water to add weight can help.

How to play:

•Start by standing up straight, shoulders touching your earlobes and shrugging.

• Elbows should also be straight and hands should be on the sides of the thighs. You don't have to turn your shoulders to do this. A shrug is enough.

7. Front lift: The next chest exercise uses dumbbells in both hands. By moving the arms up and down independently, this exercise strengthens the shoulder muscles and tones the chest.

Implementation steps:

• The reach of your hands should be shoulder height and this time your arms should be parallel to the floor.

• So you don't have to worry about keeping your elbows away from your hands or higher than that for recording. This exercise is easier and can be done easily twice a day.

8. Side Lift: The side raise is a great exercise to reduce the excess fat around your breasts and reduce the size by a few inches. Using a dumbbell can increase the effectiveness of this exercise for faster results. In addition to firmer breasts, you may also notice a slight improvement in your figure. Implementation steps:

• Start by keeping an upright position, then place your palms facing your thighs.

•Make sure your elbows are straight and far apart;

Raise your arms so that they are parallel to the floor.

• Repeat 5 times, but remember to pause for 10 seconds each time before starting the next set. This is one of the powerful breast reduction exercises with no side effects.

ADDITIONAL TIPS FOR REDUCING BREAST SIZE NATURALLY:

Unless you have large breasts that require surgery, you can try these tips to reduce your breast size at home:

• Exercise regularly. There is no shortcut to success, including the removal of excess fat from the chest area. • In addition to a targeted exercise plan, eat a healthy diet rich in fiber, vitamins and minerals.

• keep a check on your calories and maintain a good body mass index.

• Make sure your metabolism is on track. Fast digestion is essential for burning calories.

• Finally, avoid clothes that can make you look taller

. Wearing a shrink bra can temporarily fix your problem and make it appear one size down. So women! Before the problem becomes too uncomfortable, you must try these best exercises to reduce breast size. You will not only see an improvement in bust size but also gain an overall toned body. To see visible results, you must promise yourself to exercise regularly and maintain a healthy lifestyle.

Note: In cases of trying breast reduction exercises at home, you can also get advice from your doctor.

HOW TO REDUCE YOUR BREAST SIZE QUICKLY.

By doing cardio and other exercises as well as pushups and chest presses which consumes fewer calories than you burn, you can reduce your bust size. You can also add flax seed and ginger to your diet for faster results. This is how to reduce your breast size in one day. Although large breasts may seem embarrassing, they can cause severe and persistent back pain. Try these simple exercises to reduce breast size easily! Breast reduction is important for your general well-being, considering the constant muscle tension in your shoulders, neck and back leading to stabbing pains. After reducing your breast size and you do not want it to be known by your associates, onefeng triangle silicone breast form mastectomy prosthesis concave bra enhancer may be better option for you.

WHAT CAUSES BIGGER BREASTS?

Breast size is often determined by a combination of genetic and hormonal factors. One of the reasons is that hormonal changes can cause breast growth in the human body. In addition to hormonal factors, an unhealthy and moderate lifestyle that leads to weight gain also affects breast size. Other factors that cause breasts to grow are:-

> menstrual cycle
> Obesity
> Polycystic ovary
> Pregnancy
> Breast feeding
> Breast lumps

> Hereditary
> Hormone therapy
> Abortions
> Infections
> Medications
> Breast cancer
> surgery

During puberty or pregnancy, estrogen and progesterone levels in the body increase significantly, thereby causing breast development. This leads to an increase in breast size and number of ducts. In some women, the breasts become abnormally large, heavy, and painful. Hence, breast enlargement can be in natural or cosmetic form.

THE BEST WAY TO REDUCE BREASTS SIZE NATURALLY:-

The frequently ask question is, how can I make my breasts smaller without exercise? We understand how bigger breast can be heavy, a times it looks like a burden but the following natural drinks can be of help to reduce breasts size:-

1. Fenugreek -You need 3 tablespoons of fenugreek seeds with Water. What you need to do is:-

- ❖ Soak 3 tablespoons of fenugreek seeds overnight.
- ❖ Grind them the next day to make a thick paste.
- ❖ Apply this mixture evenly on both your breasts.

❖ **Then rinse and dry.**

How often - 2-4 times a week.

How it works?

Anecdotal evidence shows that fenugreek seeds can prevent sagging, improve breast firmness, and reduces breast size.

2. Flaxseed You will need 1 tablespoon ground flaxseed and 1 glass of warm water. What you need to do is:-

❖ **Mix ingredients and drinks.**

❖ **Alternatively, you can also add flax seed meal to your favorite dish or juice. This hormone controls the growth of the milk ducts in the breasts. Therefore,** the consumption of flaxseeds may have some effect in reducing breast size.

3. Ginger- You will need 1 teaspoon of grated ginger, 1 cup of water and 1 teaspoon of honey.

What you need to do is:-

- ❖ Boil grated ginger for 1minute and filter the water.
- ❖ Let it cool.
- ❖ Add honey and drink 3 times daily.

How does it work?

Regular ginger consumption helps control obesity and may contribute to weight loss and associated risks. This can have an overall impact on your body weight and help improve sagging breasts. Ginger tea is very good for breast reduction with no side effects. Ginger has oxidants that have been proven to be effective for breast reduction.

For faster result on how to reduce your breast size in one day, mix ginger with lime in hot water and drink.

If you want to substitute honey in your tea, agave nectar is a great substitute.

4. Green tea you will need

- 1 teaspoon of green tea

- 1 cup of water

- 1 teaspoon of honey

What you should do is:-

* ❖ **Boil the tea leaves for 1 minute and filter the water.**
* ❖ **Cool, add honey and drink.**
* ❖ **Drink 3 times a day.**

How effective?

Green tea can help reduce body weight and body mass index. Weight gain is one of the causes of enlarged glands. Therefore, reducing body weight can help reduce breast size.

5. You need neem and turmeric

* **Neem leaves**

* **2 teaspoons of turmeric powder**

* **2 glasses of water**

* **1 teaspoon of honey**

What to do is:-

- ❖ Boil neem leaves for 2-3 minutes and filter the water.
- ❖ Add turmeric and honey and drink. How long Once a day.

How it works?

This remedy is especially helpful if you are trying to lose breast fat after pregnancy or breastfeeding. Internal inflammation is associated with obesity and fat deposition. Turmeric and neem helps your body to overcome inflammations. These help reduce breast size.

6. Garcinia Cambogia (Malabar Me)
You need • 200-500 mg of garcinia cambogia supplement if you must Consume 200-500 mg of garcinia

cambogia supplement after consulting your doctor. Frequently 3 times a day or as recommended by your doctor.

How it works

Garcinia cambogia supplement can lose weight, it helps in overall weight management and obesity, and also helps reduce breast size. However, supplementation alone may not help. You must exercise to lose weight.

7. Fish oil- You need fish oil supplement (1000mg) what should you do is:-

 Take fish oil supplements as suggested. It also helps to reduce breast size due to pregnancy or weight gain. However, supplements alone may not help with weight loss. You need exercise to maintain a healthy weight.

Note, do not consume any nutritional supplements without consulting your doctor.

8. Spinach -you will need, • 2-3 bunches of spinach.

 What you need to do is:-

1. Make a spinach smoothie with almond milk and berries, drink daily.

TIPS ON HOW TO REDUCE YOUR BREAST SIZE.

1. Massage the breasts to reduce fat deposits within the breast tissue.

2. Choose a bra that fits your size and supports your breasts. An ill-fitting bra can do more harm than good. Also, avoid wearing it for a long period of time, and replace it after 6 months (after 180 uses).

3. Increase your water intake and stay hydrated to reduce fat accumulation in your body. This keeps the skin elastic and also prevents the breasts from sagging.

4. Consult a nutritionist and follow a diet that meets your body's needs to

maintain overall health and weight and ultimately reduce breast size.

FOODS THAT CAN REDUCE BREASTS SIZE

A high body mass index and weight gain directly affect breast size. So maintain a proper diet and an optimal body mass index in order to reduce your breast size. Please consult a nutritionist or dietician for the proper breast reduction diet chart for your body type and needs. Start by including these foods in your diet:

• Nuts

• Leafy Vegetables

• Ginger

• Garlic

• Citrus Fruits

- **Honey**

- **Tomatoes**

- **Red Meat**

- **Whole Grains**

Also, avoid fried and processed foods. Or take it in moderation.

A healthy diet is beneficial when combined with exercise. Eating the right foods plays an important role in how much fat is stored in the body and overall body fat can contribute to breast size.

By following a quantitatively balanced diet that is, calculating calories combined with exercise, you will not only contribute to weight loss, but also reduce your bust size. Simple and regular exercises at home will help you reduce your bust size. One can tone the pectoral muscles well, thereby giving a beautiful figure and a toned body.

HOW TO REDUCE BREASTS SIZE DURING AND AFTER PREGNANCY.

During and after pregnancy, the breasts may increase in size. Breasts tend to grow during pregnancy and remain large while they are breastfeeding. The increase in size is especially noticeable in the first few weeks after giving birth, as breast milk supply is still regulating itself.

Along with milk production and hormonal effects, people also put on body fat during pregnancy, some of which gets deposited in the breast tissues making it fuller.

Many people find that their breasts slowly shrink as they lose pregnancy weight, and others find that their breasts remain slightly larger after having a baby.

How to reduce breast milk during or after pregnancy and breastfeeding is by eating healthy diets.

Consult your doctor about any concerns that may arise.

WHAT CAUSES BREAST PAINS?

Breast pains are common during menstrual cycle. Learn the different types of breast pains and when to see a doctor. If natural solutions don't work, you can opt for breast reduction surgery which is usually done in a hospital and takes a few hours with a relatively longer recovery time. This procedure involves removing fat, skin, and tissue from the lower part of the breast. Alternatively, you can opt for other non-surgical alternatives, such as breast reduction pills and breast reduction creams that are said to reduce breast size. How to reduce breast size in 1 week or how to reduce breast fats are common questions that medical professionals receive. You can maintain the look and shape of your breasts if you follow an active and fit lifestyle. Your breast size is affected by many factors such as age and body mass index. You can improve sagging and reduce breast size by following simple home remedies without the high cost of breast reduction like surgery. These remedies contain ingredients that promote skin firmness or may help with weight loss. These properties can help improve the overall appearance of your breasts. Follow a nutritious diet and regular exercise program for optimal results. Consult your healthcare provider about the use of braces and support bras that can help improve your appearance.

CAN LARGE BREASTS BE REDUCED?

For women with large breasts, breast reduction surgery can reduce discomfort and improve appearance. Breast reduction can also help improve self-image and improve the ability to participate in physical activity.

Will my breasts naturally shrink?

Breasts are usually made up of a combination of fatty and fibrous tissue. Adipose tissue can be reduced through exercise and diet, but fibrous tissue cannot. This is why some people succeed with natural remedies and others do not.

Surgical breast reduction produces better results for many patients, but diet and exercise can also have noticeable results. However, breast reduction and weight loss with a healthy lifestyle is often more difficult than people realize. When diet and exercise alone are not enough to reduce breast size, many people turn to cosmetic procedures such as breast reduction and liposuction.

However, those who are determined to avoid breast reduction surgery need not lose hope, as many women are able to reduce fat levels naturally, especially in the breasts. This is made possible by a healthy lifestyle that includes a nutritious diet and regular exercise, which can lead to overall weight loss.

However, due to the unique structure of the breast, it may not be possible to reduce breast size despite diet and exercise. Breasts are usually composed of a combination of adipose and fibrous tissue. Adipose tissue can be reduced through exercise and diet, but fibrous tissue cannot. This is why some grow naturally and others do not, because breast tissue contains more fibrous tissue than fatty tissue, cosmetic procedures may be the best option for those who cannot achieve noticeable results with diet and exercise alone. Breast reduction surgery reduces the overall size of the breast, leaving a limited scar that is hidden and virtually undetectable. Reducing overly large breasts provides patients with many benefits, including: you will feel less pain in your neck and shoulders and an overall feeling of fatigue.

If traditional natural methods prove ineffective, contact your doctor about breast reduction and to schedule an appointment.

HOW TO REDUCE BREAST: NATURAL AND SURGERY METHODS.

Can you reduce breast size without surgery? Having full breasts is not always desirable. In fact, having large and heavy breasts can be a real pain for many women, causing chronic back, neck and shoulder problems or unwanted looks. If you want nothing more than to have smaller, lighter breasts, all you want is to do it without surgery. Understandably, breast reduction surgery is a big step forward. However, although cosmetic treatments are making great strides on faces and body surgeries, we are yet to find safe and effective surgery solutions to bigger breast.

Breasts continue to develop throughout a woman's life. Some women get frustrated that they have always had big breasts, or that their breasts have become larger due to pregnancy or weight gain. In some cases, some women consider large breasts to be an aesthetic or cosmetic advantage, but many women have problems with large breasts because of shoulder, neck and back pains they usually encountered. The Side effects associated with all general surgical procedures are applicable. This includes the following items.

- **Risks of anesthesia**

- Allergy to dressings, sutures, glues, blood products, topical medications or injections

- Infection

- Bleeding (hematoid)

- Poor wound healing

- Pain near the incision site

- Scars

Also, there are some side effects specific to this type of surgery that you should also be aware of.

- Changes in sensation in the nipple or breast, which may be temporary or permanent

- Breast asymmetry

- Abnormal breast shape

• **Possible surgical correction**

• **Irregular breast firmness**

• **None ability to breastfeed**

• **Possible loss of breast skin/tissue where the incisions meet.**

• **Partial loss of nipple and areola These risk and side effects are very common. However, you should talk to your doctor and ask any questions you may have before the procedure for peace of mind.**

If you have tried all of the above natural methods without seeing results, breast reduction surgery may be the best option for you. You should talk to your plastic surgeon about your body goals.

WHAT IS THE COST OF BREAST REDUCTION SURGERY?

The cost of breast reduction surgery depends on many different factors. Some of these factors include individual doctor or surgeon fees, surgery center location, anesthesia fees, and more. Be sure to discuss the cost of surgery before making a final decision with your doctor. Remember that insurance usually does not cover cosmetic surgery. However, in the case of breast reduction, insurance may cover the costs. If you're having breast reduction surgery for health reasons, talk to your doctor about how to make sure your insurance covers your costs. Doctors offer financial plans for patients, so be sure to ask. Finding the Right Plastic Surgeon to Reduce Breast Size After trying all natural methods with no results may be your best bet. During your first consultation, the right plastic surgeon will address all of your concerns regarding surgery and recovery. He or she will also make sure to answer any lingering questions about the process that will help you feel as comfortable as possible. It is important that you find a doctor who will respect your decision and will reassure you of safe operation and quick recovery processes. If you are not convince when talking to your doctor, then get a second opinion. This can be important in making the most informed medical decisions possible.

STEPS TO REDUCE BREAST SIZE?

There are many reasons why you might want to reduce your breast size. Over time, large breasts can lead to serious problems such as back pain, poor posture, and difficulty in breathing. In addition, large breasts tend to sag more with age. If you have large breasts and want to change, start with the steps below to know how to reduce your breast size:-

1. Have fewer calories. In order to lose weight, you need fewer calories. Calories are our body's fuel

and when we consume fewer calories, the body will start burning fat. This can be achieved with a slight mix of activity level and diet. This fewer calories deficit is only for temporal. Once you have reached your goal weight, you will need to adjust your calorie intake to your activity level.

2. Reduce eating sugar, salt and fatty foods. Start by minimizing the amount of salt, unhealthy fats, and sugar in your diet. Salt holds water in the body and causes bloating, sugar is an inefficient calorie that makes you hungry. Salt is found in canned soups, many meats mainly hot dogs, salami, bacon, pizza, chips, and many other foods. Eating

of salt should be less than 100 mg a day. However, do not stop completely. Salt is needed for the body to function properly, especially when you start exercising. Sugar is found naturally in candy, but it can also be found in many commercial coffees such as Starbucks, soft drinks, and fruit juices.

3. Eating too much fruit will add sugar! Unhealthy fats include trans-fats and saturated fats found in red meat, butter, mayonnaise, and fried foods. Healthy fats, such as unsaturated and polyunsaturated fats, are healthy and can be found in foods like fish and nuts. Eat nutritious foods.

4. Eating nutrient-rich foods naturally makes you feel full even when you eat less. Switching to fruits and vegetables is not enough. There are many differences between celery stalks and broccoli.

5. Nutritious grains include oatmeal, quinoa, barley, and brown rice. When buying bread, be sure to buy whole grain bread instead of multi-grain bread. Whole grains are the healthier choice of the two, and white bread offers fewer nutritional benefits than multigrain breads. Nutritious vegetables and fruits include lemons, cranberries, bananas, spinach, broccoli, asparagus, and Brussels sprouts. The best sources of protein are

chicken, fish, eggs, nuts and beans. They are low in unhealthy fats and still contain the protein you need for your daily energy and exercise routine. Dairy products include low-fat plain yogurt flavored with fresh fruit, cheese, and low-fat milk. Notes, don't only eat food, but also have a clean, healthy and balanced diet.

6. Wear a tight sports bra. A high-quality sports bra with maximum support example fruit of the loom women's spaghetti strap cotton pull over sports bra.It is probably the easiest way to hold your bust and shrink it in the most comfortable way, buy these from reputable brands for maximum effectiveness.

Low-quality sports bras wear out quickly and lose their effectiveness.

7. Wear a correct size of bra. You can also buy regular bras that can "shrink" your breasts by making them look less bulky. This is called fitted bras. Again, quality from great brands is on your side. However, these primarily work only for busts in the C-DD range.

8. For a good breast posture, avoid wearing clothes like ceboyel women criss cross sexy summer tops halter neck tank tops without bra.

9. Make sure you are wearing an appropriate supportive bra. Just wearing the correct size minimally padded bra will give you about the

same effect as a much more expensive minimally padded bra. This is more convenient than any other option and generally good advice.

For example, it is estimated that 73% of women wear the wrong bra size so putting on the right size of bra would be best bet.

The following can are recommended while undergoing breast reduction process:-

❖ Hiplaygirl silicone breast forms- waterdrop prosthesis crossdressers mastectomy A-GG cup.

❖ **Brabic shaper tops for women arm compression front closure bra tank shapewear.**

❖ **Drain holder after tummy tuck mastectomy drain holder for shower breast reduction, recovery must have drainage pouch tube pockets.**

❖ **Wear vollence strap on silicone breast forms fake boobs, it is so lovely even crossdressers wear it.**

10. Try a chest tie. If you're really desperate and other options don't work, try tying your breasts. Consider buying a safe chest binder for transgender people.

Whatever you use, don't bind for more than 4-8 hours.

These tricks are for women working on how to reduce cup size from d to b and perfect for anyone wearing a US B-DD cup. Anything larger than this is unlikely to leave a large dent.

10. Don't wear cloth that makes you uncomfortable. Of course, you should never allow cosmetics to influence your style of clothing.

You have the right to dress your way, but small adjustments can make a big difference in how your breasts look.

❖ Make sure you choose the right clothes, not too tight or too big.

❖ **Cuts that accentuate the bust should also be avoided. B. Items with a natural waist, cowl neck tops, or tops with pleats or gathers at the bust.**

❖ **Emphasize on hips instead of these elements, it will make your breasts look smaller in size.**

THE BREASTS REDUCTION CREAMS

Below are some of the best breast reduction creams that are readily available and safe to use.

1. VLCC Shape Up Breast Reduction/Firming Cream:

This brand is so popular when we talk about women and their body care, it is also known as every woman's desire. VLCC Shape up is one of such breast reduction cream that provides firmness to it. They claim that you will start seeing the results on or before 21 days. VLCC Breast Reduction cream is ayurvedic which is made up of organic and natural ingredients. So next time you want someone to envy your good looks and perfect figure, this is it!

The key Ingredients: Oils of Simmondsia California (Jojoba) 0.5%, Vitis Vinifera Seed (Grape Seed)0.3%, Cyperus Pertenuis (Cyprus)0.15%, Rosmarinus Officinalis (Rosemary) 0.1%, Geranium Sylvaticum (Geranium) 0.2%, Punica Grantum (Pomegranate) 0.5%, Soja Hispida (Soybean) Extract 1%, Cream Base Q.S.

How To Use:

• Take an adequate quantity of cream and apply from the base of the breasts to the neck with firm and circular upward strokes.

• It helps the skin's support structure over the entire lift zone.

• Use the cream daily and allow it to remain on your body for 6-8 hours.

• Avoid applying on the nipple area.

Key Benefits are:-

> Natural Cream.
> Firms Breasts.
> It reduces sagging and oversize breasts.

2. In Life Breast Reduction Cream:

This cream works by motivating the enlargement of cells in your body. Also, the herbal formula helps to control the pH plus hydration issue in the body. By gradually boosting the number of breast tissues; it assists one to improve breast size logically. Whatever Natural herbs are included in the cream which increases fatty tissues ahead correct assimilation, thus providing reduction to your breast.

The key Ingredients are Herbal ingredients.

How To Use:

• Massage your breast gently in the upward direction and in back and forth movement to cover the entire area.

• Rub the cream and leave it for the entire day.

Key Benefits are:-

➢ It has no harmful chemicals.

- ➢ **Good packaging guaranteed.**
- ➢ **Reasonable pricing.**

3. Alexaderm Breast Reduction and Contouring Cream:

It has low Scent, Non-greasy, and no stain plus it is simple to smear. One tube is enough for giving the result. You can use it twice a day; once in the morning and other in the night. Is it possible to reduce breast size? Yes,Alexaderm is a natural cream that reduces breast size. However, with assurance, the benefits are equally eye-catching and hard to miss. It has no side effects so you need not to worry. It can be used by the teens in their growing years to effectively control the saggy breasts.

The key Ingredients are puria, glycerol, ginkgo, rhubarb cream concentrate, Aloe Vera extract, caffeine silanol, safflower oil.

How To Use:

• Use regularly according to instructions.

Key Benefits:

➢ It has good packaging.
➢ It is easy to use.
➢ It has no side effects.

4. Lasky Herbal Blossom Cream Reduces Breast Size:

It contains herbs that are beneficial in natural firmness, toning and improves the breast tissues, regulate hormones, increases the fatty tissues plus ligaments and increases blood flow. It reinforces the triangle of skin that holds the bust it called natural bra. This cream has a tapering prove that helps tone the muscle-sustaining skin. The herbal cream discussed here are different from cosmetic ones. The cream worth it price you pay and guarantee quick results because of it ingredients and the way it works.

How To Use:

• Use regularly according to
instructions.

Key Benefits:

> It contains Ayurvedic formula.
> It is safe on skin.
> It gives good and lovely shape.

The above research is done so you
can find trusted products for your
health and wellness. So do the
following for a better result:-

• Check ingredients and composition
thoroughly do they have the
potential to cause harm?

• Check with proves all health
claims whether they align with the
current body of scientific evidence.

• Diligently assess the brand and be sure it operates with integrity and adhere to industry best practices.

Using: • Use as often as directed. Main benefits are:-

• Good packaging.

• Easy to use.

• No side effects.

5. Cute Hashmi B Ice Cream: This is a natural breast reduction cream that successfully reduces breast size in tall women. It controls the levels of the hormone estrogen in women responsible for their breast size. The cream does not only reduce breast size naturally, but it has other benefits like improving

shape, toning body, increasing firmness and also preventing sagging of breasts. It is a GMP certified product created from a blend of natural herbal ingredients.

Among breast reduction creams, this one tops the list. The amount to pay is quite high but the bottle lasts a long time and there are usually no reported side effects. As if that wasn't good news, you also get great deals like reduced breast sagging and some of the same achieved with the promised cream.

6. Lass Cellulite Massage Oil: This massage oil is a special blend of essential oils combined with anti-cellulite properties. By gently

massaging the surface of the skin, it helps to eliminate extreme cellulite. It burns excess fat in the cells into expendable energy and is massaged regularly and helps you get a tighter, firmer, and slimmer waist and abdomen. This product also contains silver birch and cypress oils which have excellent anti-cellulite properties. This breast reduction cream will achieve significant positive results after regular use. Try this safe massage oil for best results.

7. Neutri-herbes Breast Firming Cream Firming Breast Shape: This breast enhancement cream contains Pueraria wild radix extract, collagen, ginseng, Xiong river

angelica, black frankincense helps to firm and reduce breast. Also, on this list is a good breast reduction cream that gives good results immediately. It is not only common among women who have different preferences about the cream they choose, but also for those who pay attention to everything that happens to their bodies.

 It has no side effects

It is clinically tested so you need not to worry.

8. Real Plus body slimming cream, Chinese herbal slimming cosmetics, breast reduction cream:

These are demineralized water, Poria, glycerol, ginkgo, concentrated

rhubarb cream, aloe extract,
caffeine silanol, safflower oil.
Slimming cream can regulate blood
circulation and burn fat quickly. It
also inhibits the fascination of body
fat; It also opens pores to release
toxins that drain out quickly. The
price of this cream is relatively
cheap since its shelf life is almost 3
years. The number of boxes varies
depending on the price, but the price
is durable.

WHAT IS GIANT BREASTS?

Macromastia, or mammary
hyperplasia, is a rare condition in
which very large breasts occur due
to excessive growth of breast
tissue. It affects those who are
assigned as female at birth. Large

breasts result in rapid, disproportionate breast growth. The rate at which breasts grow can vary from weeks to years. The tissue is most often benign (non-cancerous).

BIG BREASTS ARE CHARACTERIZED BY:

• Breasts with at least 5 pounds of excess breast tissue.

• Excess breast tissue that accounts for 3% or more of the total weight may occur during puberty, pregnancy, or from taking medications; sometimes it happens spontaneously for no reason.

Gigantomastia is also known as Macromastia. However, large breasts are defined as excess breast tissue weighing less than 5-6 pounds. Big breasts are divided into four types.

• Juvenile mammata: This type occurs during puberty.

 • Drug induced mammary gland or drug-induced: Occurs after taking certain drugs.

• Idiopathic mammary glands: The cause of mammary glands is unknown or cannot be determined. Idiopathic giant breasts are the most common form.

• Gestational macromastia: Macromastia occurs during pregnancy.

HOW COMMON IS LARGE BREASTS?

This is a rare disease. Just fewer than 300 cases have been reported.

What are the signs, symptoms and causes of large breasts?

Very large breasts can be physically and emotionally painful.

The most common symptoms of breast enlargement are:

• Infections of the breast, especially the skin under the breast.

• Neck and back pain from being pulled by the chest.

• Bad posture.

• Loss of feeling in nipples.

• Chest pain.

• **Painful and itchy bumps on the skin from bra straps.**

HOW IS IT DIAGNOSED?

Your health care provider will carry out full examination on your body; he/she must have known your health history. Your doctor will need to know how your breast size has changed, what other symptoms you have, and if you are taking any medications. No further tests are usually needed to confirm the diagnosis.

HOW TO TREAT LARGER BREASTS

There is no one-size-fits-all treatment for large breasts. You and your doctor can discuss all treatment options and weigh their risks and benefits.

Depending on the severity of the symptoms and the size of the breast, your doctor may recommend breast reduction surgery or medications to treat large breasts. If the breast enlargement recurs or is severe, your doctor may recommend a mastectomy.

Breasts size reduction can save you the stress of heaviness while undergoing that momcozy hands free pumping bra or Adjustable breast pump holding is best for you.

WHAT DRUGS CAN TREAT LARGE BREASTS?

There are drugs that can stop the growth of breast tissue. Your doctor may prescribe one of the following medicines:

• Tamoxifen.

• Medroxyprogesterone.

• Danazol.

• Bromocriptine.

In some cases, it is sufficient to slow the growth of breast tissue. In other cases, surgery should be

combined with breast reduction process.

CAN SURGERY TREAT LARGER BREASTS?

Large breasts can be treated with breast reduction surgery. A surgeon makes an incision in your chest and removes excess fat, tissue, and skin. Once the desired breast size is reached, the incision is closed with sutures. The nipple and areola may need to be repositioned to accommodate the new size and shape of the breast. The operation takes several hours and may require a long hospital stay.

Mastectomy may be recommended for severe or recurrent large breasts. The health practitioner gets rid of the complete breast.

Mastectomy carries risks and should be discussed with a doctor.

How long will it take to recover from treatment?

Expect some pain, swelling and bruising in the first few days after breast reduction. Doctors may prescribe antibiotics to prevent infection and pain relievers to relieve symptoms. A breast exam and suture removal will be scheduled at your next appointment. Most people recover and resume light activity within a week. Once the swelling subsides, your breasts will take on their final shape and size. Scars are noticeable, but most surgeons try to keep them to a minimum.

If you have a mastectomy, you will recover within a month. Your exact recovery time will vary depending on your age, medical condition, and other factors.

What complications can occur with large breasts?

Large breasts can cause:

• Neck and back pain.

• Unable to walk, run or play sports.

• Skin infections in brassieres.

• Chest pain.

• Breastfeeding Challenges.

• Skin irritation or itching.

In addition to these physical symptoms, oversized breasts can lead to psychological and social problems such as depression, anxiety, and poor body image.

Large breasts can cause problems for pregnant women, including poor fetal growth, mastitis, and low milk production.

HOW TO AVOID BREAST AUGMENTATION

There is nothing you can do to reduce the risk of breast augmentation. Researchers say the cause of breast growth is unknown.

What happens if I get this disease?

Large breasts usually do not cause serious complications. Depending on the severity of the symptoms of large breasts, everyday life can be painful and uncomfortable. Talk to your doctor about how to relieve your symptoms and whether you notice lumps or breast cancer.

CONCLUSIONS.

Larger breasts can be very inconvenience or a source of significant pains to ladies. The natural methods outlined above can help you reduce your breast size, such as losing weight and eating a healthy food. Wearing specific bras and binders can also reduce the appearance of your breast; make them look lovely and attractive.

Natural remedies for breast reduction are cost effective and do not have side effect, no pains or scars, but if you consider surgery as an option, you can consult your doctor. In a recent poll, people who had breast reduction surgery found that over 93 percent said they were satisfied with their results.

Talking about breast size can be emotional topic because of social and cultural ideas about the meaning of breasts and how people feel about their own breasts.

How to reduce breasts size through natural remedies can improve firmness and brighten your breasts.

Breasts are very sensitive to changes in weight, so it is quite common to have a cup lift after gaining a few pounds. It can put too much pressure on them, so learning about breast reduction can be beneficial in the long run. If you are trying to tighten your breasts without surgery, you can try the tips described in this book.

Health care providers understand the challenges that people with very large breasts often face and can be of help. People struggling with breast size issues or concerned about breast health can see their doctors before making significant lifestyle changes.